BIOETHICAL ISSUES

POPE JOHN PAUL II
LECTURE SERIES IN BIOETHICS
edited by
Rev. Francis J. Lescoe, Ph.D.
and
Rev. David Q. Liptak, D. Min.

. . . .

VOL. II
BIOETHICAL ISSUES
I. THE BIOLOGICAL REVOLUTION AND THE MYTH OF PROMETHEUS
by
Raymond Dennehy, Ph.D.
Professor of Philosophy, University of San Francisco

II. A CHRISTIAN ETHICS OF LIMITING MEDICAL TREATMENT: GUIDANCE FOR PATIENTS, PROXY DECISION MAKERS AND COUNSELORS
by
Germain Grisez, Ph.D.
The Reverend Harry J. Flynn *Professor of Christian Ethics Mount Saint Mary's College*

POPE JOHN PAUL II BIOETHICS CENTER
Holy Apostles College and Seminary
Cromwell, CT 06416

ISBN 0-910919-04-6

Lescoe, Francis J. and Liptak, David Q., Editors
Pope John Paul II Lecture Series in Bioethics
Vol. II
Dennehy, Raymond and Grisez, Germain
Bioethical Issues

+Daniel P. Reilly, D.D.
Bishop of Norwich
August 22, 1986

Distributors for the trade:
MARIEL PUBLICATIONS
196 Eddy Glover Boulevard
New Britain, CT 06053

ANNOUNCEMENT

The Pope John Paul II Bioethics Center has been instituted for the purpose of articulating authentic Catholic teaching with respect to medical science and technology.

In his first encyclical, Redemptor Hominis, *John Paul defended the priority of ethics over science and technology:*

> *The development of technology and the development of contemporary civilization, which is marked by the ascendancy of technology, demand a proportional development of morals and ethics. (Section 16)*

Today, with an unprecedented rush of scientific discoveries and technological breakthroughs, this priority is being doubted, ignored and challenged. Traditional Christian principles repeatedly affirmed by the Church's magisterium, have been set aside for consequentialism, behaviorism, relativism, context morality, secularism and other inadequate or erroneous theories in misleading, false and sometimes inane attempts to address ethically fresh scientific insights or revolutionary technological advances.

The purpose of this Center is twofold. First, we shall endeavor to impart to our seminarians, here at Holy Apostles College and Seminary, a solid foundation in medical ethics and bioethical science. Secondly, we shall share our investigations and findings by publishing periodic monographs, in addition to the annual Pope John Paul II Lectures in Bioethics.

THE POPE JOHN PAUL II LECTURES
IN BIOETHICS
HAVE BEEN MADE POSSIBLE THROUGH
THE GENEROSITY OF
REVEREND LEO J. KINSELLA
OUR LADY OF THE SNOWS
CHICAGO, ILLINOIS

TABLE OF CONTENTS

I. THE BIOLOGICAL REVOLUTION AND THE MYTH OF PROMETHEUS
by Raymond Dennehy

INTRODUCTION

Next to the scientific revolution itself, the biological revolution is the greatest of all the purely human revolutions thus far. I say "purely human revolutions" because the greatest of all revolutions was that effected by Christianity. But since the latter consisted of Christ entering human history, it was revolution by Divine intervention and therefore belongs in a class by itself. I shall, however, have occasion to advert to the significance of Christianity for the biological revolution later in this presentation. The magnitude of the biological revolution originates in the fact that it signals a decisive breakthrough in our mastery over *internal* nature. While the other revolutions, such as the Industrial Revolution, were confined in their influence to man's environment, advances in the biological sciences bring with them the promise of manipulating his own being even unto the point of manufacturing human beings in his own image. The generation of human life by in vitro fertilization will soon be a commonplace as well as will be the storage of frozen human embryos. Although other projects frequently discussed, such as recombining DNA, other forms of genetic engineering, and cloning remain very far from application to human beings, their very prospect confronts us with the question, "What Sort of People Should There Be?"[1] Speculations, however fantastic, such as the creation of computers with human brains (cyborgs) and computers with biological parts capable of replacing themselves,[2] are "thought experiments"[3] sufficiently fascinating to challenge our conception of human nature.

As we might have expected, secular humanism cannot conceal an enthusiasm for the biological revolution, despite expressions of concern from some of its advocates about mismanagement and violations of liberty. No doubt, the temptation to refashion man so that he will be perfect manifests itself today *genetically* as opposed to its former

7

political manifestation. Classical political theory — e.g., as set forth by Plato, Aristotle, Augustine, and Aquinas — saw temporal society as the "second best state" whose task was to mitigate by law and custom human imperfection insofar as it asserted the impossibility of attaining perfect justice in this life.[4] But modern political theory, since Marsilius of Padua, has rejected as irrelevant to man's temporal political projects the supratemporal concerns of religion, such as heaven and hell. It was accordingly inevitable that modern political theorists should have found themselves with no alternative than that of seeking the ultimate reward and punishment in temporal society alone: human perfection will be attainable in this life or not at all. Given this outlook, it is hardly surprising that biological manipulation, dangling before the world the rich promises of genetic engineering, should now vie with political control as the preeminent instrument for the eradication of "evil" from human conduct and for making man perfect.[5]

But the biological revolution has a more fundamental significance than as an extension of the ambitions of modern political theory. Nowhere is this significance more powerfully expressed than in the Myth of Prometheus. The common version of the myth tells of *Prometheus pyrphoros*, who stole fire (the symbol of culture) from Zeus and gave it to man. The other version, which probably had a different and later origin, tells of *Prometheus plasticator*, who creates man.[6] Obviously, the second version is simply a specific amplification of the aspirations expressed in the older version. The Promethean figure may be described as one who is constantly striving to unlock the secrets of nature and who refuses to acknowledge any limits to the human mind's capacity to understand them. Such an individual might even covet the knowledge of God. This rebellion against human limitation emerges quite clearly in Goethe's *Faust*. The afflatus for Faust's lifelong pursuit of learning was not wisdom but the desire to be like God:

> I, the image of godhead, who thought myself near to the mirror of eternal truth, enjoyed myself in heaven's clear radiance and stripped of all mortality; I, more than a cherub, I, whose free strength already dream-

ed it flowed through the veins of nature and dared
presume to enjoy the creative life of the gods — I must
do penance for that.[7]

It would therefore be mistaken to categorize the Promethean figure simply in terms of expanding the frontiers
of human knowledge, discovering the philosopher's stone,
or even sharing the Divine wisdom. The Promethean *elan*
drives some human beings to become creators of human
life itself. Consider, for example, the homunculus aspired
to by Paracelsus,[8] the creation of an homunculus by Wagner
in Part Two of *Faust* [9] and the Frankenstein monster in Mary
Shelley's novel, appropriately subtitled *The Modern Prometheus* .[10]

It is clear that the biological revolution expresses the Promethean myth in contemporary terms. It is Promethean not
only insofar as it testifies to man's relentless striving to
enlarge his knowledge but also insofar as it testifies to his
desire to increase his domination over the universe — even
into the creation of human life itself.

To be sure, the Promethean myth enshrines man's
preeminence in nature, his nobility as a seeker of truth and
self-determining agent. But we should not allow its positive
side to blind us to its down side. The Promethean myth is
a tragedy: Prometheus is monstrously punished for bringing fire and hope to mankind. Disaster ineluctably follows
from the attempt to emulate God. Wagner's homunculus
dashes itself to bits on the rocks; the Frankenstein monster
enslaves and destroys its creator but only after inflicting suffering and death on innocent people.

But the Promethean need not be a tragic figure. Man's
desire for increasing knowledge of and domination over
nature are the springs of human progress. The Promethean
tragedy presupposes a rivalry between God and man
(despite allusions to a future reconciliation in Aeschylus'
Promethean Bound), e.g., *Promethean Bound, Faust,* and
Frankenstein; it would not be inappropriate to include here
the account of the Fall of *Genesis*. Christianity, however, rid
the myth of the rivalry. According to its teachings, God not
only made man in His own image and likeness but,
through Christ's death and resurrection, enabled him to

become His adopted son. The universe and heaven itself henceforth were his inheritance. For example, St. Albert the Great was a Promethean figure who saw man's quest for knowledge as an unfolding of God's plan. For him the honor and glory of God were the primary inspiration for the pursuit of knowledge. Enthusiastically, relentlessly, Albert pursued knowledge in theology, philosophy, the natural sciences, mathematics, and even in astrology and magic.[11] And although the intellectual appetite of his brilliant pupil, St. Thomas Aquinas, was not so broad and exotic, he too doggedly and optimistically pursued the truth wherever it might lead. Thus the sense of man's preeminent dignity implied in Prometheus' defiance of Zeus has been affirmed and superelevated by divine grace; the latter has similarly validated the desire for knowledge, power, and autonomy.

But in secular humanism — which can only be understood as a post-Christian humanism — a newer Prometheanism has arisen that is as defiant of God as it is dismissive of Him; more than an atheism, secular humanism has justly been called an "antitheism."[12] This new brand of Prometheanism has an optimism to match its enormous defiance of God. Consider, for example, Shelley's *Promethean Unbound* and Marxist doctrine. Thus two kinds of Prometheanism can be detected at work in the contemporary world. The one may be called "Christian Prometheanism" in that it manifests itself in man's insatiable desire for knowledge of and mastery over nature, but it sees the fulfilling of this desire as an unfolding of the Divine plan and its actual and final fulfillment in God alone. The preeminence of man in nature which this kind of Prometheanism presupposes derives its special *elan* from the conception of him as made in the image and likeness of God and as superelevated through divine grace to being an adopted son of God for whom the universe is now his patrimony. The second kind of Prometheanism can be called "Post-Christian Prometheanism," for although rejecting Christianity and, for that matter the existence of a supreme being, its prodigious energy and optimism presuppose the aforesaid Christian contributions.

****

Now the first point I wish to unfold in this lecture is that the biological revolution gravely threatens the future of mankind because it derives much of its impetus from Post-Christian Prometheanism. This form of Prometheanism returns man to the tradition wherein Prometheus destroys himself. The rejection of God only further conduces to the absolutizing of scientific knowledge and hardening of the dogma of infinite progress, both of which produce a deformed conception of human dignity and destiny. The inevitable result of this deformity will be the manufacture of Frankenstein monsters rather than the anticipated improvement of the human species.

The second point I wish to unfold is that the biological revolution itself is not the threat. Were Christian Prometheanism the driving force behind it, the Promethean *elan* would be channeled so as to produce an improvement in the human species as genuine as it would be spectacular. The banks of this channel would be formed, on the one side, by the realization that divine knowledge is the paradigm for knowledge, and, on the other side, by an authentic conception of man's dignity and destiny.

The destructive potential of the biological revolution warns us that man's ontological reach exceeds his ontological grasp. But the *elan* of post-Christian Prometheanism induces in man a forgetfulness of his creaturehood and intrinsic limitation. Secular humanism's failure to see that creaturehood is not a condition that can be overcome blinds its apostles to the insuperable obstacles in their path. The attendant failure to see that human power and knowledge — the two areas of Promethean endeavor — are accordingly limited and to see in what ways they are limited explains at the outset the inevitably destructive end of any Prometheanism that would rival God. Specifically, post-Christian Prometheanism unwittingly treats *power* and *knowledge* as univocal rather than analogous concepts.

I
Creature and Creator
The idea of endless progress is a modern contribution to the Promethean myth and it vividly portrays the erroneous

view of creaturehood entertained by post-Christian Prometheanism. The idea of endless progress presupposes a
lineal rather than a cyclical view of history, a view
characteristic of the Enlightenment. I think that it is
arguable that the view has its seeds in the Judeo-Christian
teachings, specifically in the doctrine that God created the
work *ex nihilo* and in the doctrine of Christ's transforma-
tion of the world through His death and resurrection:
"Behold, I have made all things new."[13] The pagan doctrine
of the eternity of the world left no room for novelty insofar
as its view of history was inevitably cyclical. For in an eternal universe — since by definition it has no beginning —
nothing new can occur; every event occurs an infinite
number of times. But if you accept the doctrine that the
world was created in time, then — since the world was new,
i.e., has a beginning — you cannot deny the possibility of
novelty and uniqueness in it, for its history must then be
lineal. This is not to say that its lineal progress must be
uninterrupted. It can have cyclical, even regressive
episodes of considerable duration and still be progressive
in its overall configuration. Nevertheless, although the
writers of the Enlightenment inherited the idea of progress
from the Judeo-Christian tradition, the idea received a new
twist at the hands of secular humanism. The Judeo-
Christian tradition can easily be harmonized with the idea
of endless progress, if by the latter is meant that human
culture will continue to advance as long as mankind exists
and that, no matter how long that may be, its approach to
perfection will always be asymptotic; that is to say, it will
never have exhausted all possibilities for improvement. For
as remarked earlier, the Judeo-Christian view is that man
cannot satisfy his desire for the infinite until he is with God
in eternity. But modern secular humanism maintains, on
the contrary, that the promises of progress can be realiz-
ed, fully and perfectly, in this temporal existence. You have
only to consider the writings of Karl Marx for an example
of this view.

Some thinkers go farther than this, maintaining that man
will continue to progress until he himself becomes God.

This view was unabashedly advanced in the nineteenth century, as can be seen in Shelley's epic poem, *Prometheus Unbound*[14] and in Feuerbach's *The Essence of Christianity*.[15] While it is far from clear what it means to say that mankind will become God, those who entertain this view regard God as a projection of human aspiration, an ideal of perfection which motivates human beings in their struggles on this earth. Feuerbach is the best known and no doubt the most influential proponent of the man-God thesis. As it goes well beyond Christ's exhortation, "Be-ye perfect as your heavenly Father is perfect," it is reasonable to ask for the rationale behind the man-god aspiration. In Feuerbach we find a rather crude materialism as the underlying reason and, indeed, it is hard to see what else could lead to so grandiose a conclusion as that man will become God. With an almost cavalier argumentation, he asserts the identity of reality with matter.[16] His materialism accordingly leads him to construe the difference between the finite and the infinite as a difference in quantity: man, the individual, is infinite; his powers are limited, making him dependent on other human beings. Mankind, on the other hand, is infinite because the totality of individual men overcomes all limitation insofar as the limitation of the powers of any individual member is completed by the powers of all the other members.[17]

The crudity of Feuerbach's philosophizing evinces itself in this wholly unsatisfactory view of what constitutes the difference between the finite and the infinite. By definition the individual is finite because to be an individual is to be set apart from others and hence to be limited. But to suppose, as Feuerbach clearly does, that the infinite is the sum total of individual parts is to fail spectacularly in understanding the meaning of "finite" and "infinite." All the men and women who ever lived could not constitute an infinity, even in numbers. For infinite is by definition what is in principle or nature unlimited. But no matter how many human beings you may imagine or wish to posit, you will never have an infinity, for you can then still imagine one more human being. No matter how stupendous the total intelligence of mankind, you can always imagine an increase in that intelligence; the same can be said of talent, power, etc.

The difference between the finite and the infinite has nothing to do with quantity *as such*, the latter being the measure of matter. The difference between them is the difference between the contingent and the necessary, between participated being and being itself. Permit me to illustrate the point by borrowing an analogy from Thomas Aquinas: if whiteness were a subsisting reality, there could only be one whiteness in existence since it would be infinite; you cannot, after all, increase the whiteness of whiteness itself. But even though there could only be one existent whiteness, there could nevertheless be many white things, for rather than being whiteness itself; i.e., white by essence, the latter only participate in whiteness. Equally, because God is existence itself, His being is infinite. Other beings, which is to say, creatures, can exist, but only because they are not, could not be, existence itself; rather they only participate in existence. Thus, no matter how vast the magnitude of its achievements, mankind can never overcome its finitude, conquer its essential limitedness, for finitude, as we have just seen, has, in principle, nothing to do with quantity and, *a fortiori*, cannot be transformed into infinitude by an increase in quantity. The totality of human beings is just as finite as one individual human being.

The failure to grasp the difference between the finite and the infinite, whether this failure be enshrined in explicit philosophical assertions or remain implicit in an ideology of unending progress and the perfectibility of man, is, I suspect, a powerful contributing factor in the conviction that man can become like God in knowledge and power. And because the conviction springs from a fundamental philosophical error, it can remain nothing more than an illusion. But, as Dostoyevsky's character Kirillov dramatically illustrates by his philosophically motivated suicide, [18] when man thinks that he himself is God, he destroys himself.

Creative Power As An Analogous Concept

The Faustian and Frankenstein examples of the Promethean figure, stretching to its limits the desire to be like God, not only conclude that the products of human creation are inferior to those of nature but also that, even though man might gain the power to control it; indeed, his very creation will turn to his own destruction. The metaphysical source of this limitation seems to have been adumbrated by Mary Shelley in the introduction to the 1831 edition of *Frankenstein*:

> . . . invention it might be humbly admitted, does not consist in creating out of a void, but out of chaos; the materials must, in the first place, be afforded: it can give form to dark, shapeless substances, but cannot bring into being the substance itself.[19]

Being a creature, man is a *creator* only analogously. While it is correct to describe Verdi as a creative composer of opera — hence his claim to the title "the Father of modern opera" — the fact remains that there could have been no Verdi (as "the Father of modern opera") if there had not first been a Bellini to influence him. And despite Newton's powerful creative genius, he would not have arrived at his theory of gravitation had he been isolated from the work of his predecessors and contemporaries.[20] Thus man, the creator, creates only analogously rather than absolutely because he does not, cannot, create *ex nihilo*; he requires preexisting materials. His "creations" can be likened to the production of a mosaic, wherein the artist arranges preexisting materials in novel ways. But even the extent of the novelty is limited by the inherent determinations and limitations of the materials. (Moreover, the novelty itself is not novel in the absolute sense, for it has for eternity been a possibility in the mind of God.) Thus man from the very start of his enterprise lacks complete control over the products of these enterprises. Faust, for example, was forced to acknowledge the limitations of his creatureliness when, having been terrified by the momentary apparition of the spirit he had conjured, he says: "If I have the power to draw you, I have no strength to hold you."[21]

The desire to be like God can have no bounds other than those of desire itself. We have noted that in the theistic universe, man's desire to attain absolute knowledge and power has its fulfillment not in this temporal life but in the Beatific Vision of the afterlife. Since the denial of God's existence does not extinguish the desire to be godlike, the atheist seeks fulfillment of this desire in temporal life. Thus the prospect of genetic engineering and cloning, both conferring on man the power to make humans as we deem desirable and the preeminent achievement, creating human life itself, thereby making him master of life and death, are crucial steps toward the fulfillment of these ultimate desires. The desire to be like God and the primordial determinations of the preexistent universe thus confront each other in what may fairly be described as mortal combat.

Knowledge As An Analogous Notion

Descartes has justly been accused of "angelizing" man by defining him simply as a thinking being. [22] But he is also guilty of deifying man by implicitly taking human knowledge as the standard of all knowing. For insofar as he refused to accept as philosophically true any proposition that cannot be apprehended as clear and distinct or demonstrated as necessarily true, he rendered intellectually suspect the highest function of intellect, namely, that whereby the human intellect apprehends truly but hazily not only the most intelligible and loftiest truths but also the concrete singular existents in their singularity. The impact of this approach to knowing on subsequent Western culture has been enormous. It has glorified human intellect and knowing, with all their limitations, as the standards. Accordingly knowing seen as an analogous notion, with Divine knowing as the primary analogate, became less and less appreciated. The current widespread view that that alone constitutes authentic knowledge which can be expressed in concepts, and in concepts of a quantitative and measurable knowledge at that, should hardly surprise us.

How this implicitly assumed notion of knowledge pertains to the biological revolution discloses itself in the eugenic ambitions of those who support the laboratory manipulation of human life. There can be little doubt that procedures such as in vitro fertilization, artificial insemination, embryo transplants, surrogate mothers, genetic engineering, and cloning excite the greatest enthusiasm among members of the scientific community and intelligentsia when seen in terms of their eugenic possibilities: the artificial production of human beings according to certain types which are regarded as desirable for the species. But this eugenic goal would reduce man to the level of brute animals, for it implies that he is primarily a *what* rather than a *who*. We value an animal primarily according to the type to which it conforms — disposition, sturdiness, fecundity, etc. In contrast, we value a human being primarily for his selfhood, for his uniqueness as a center of conscious, autonomous being. If human rights mean anything, they mean that he possesses that kind of value. For what do rights presuppose if not that individual men and women are naturally and justly entitled to live and act free from interference in certain areas of their lives? And what, in the end, can be the rationale for this entitlement but that each human being is a person or a self?

The generation of life involves the uniting of the contributed male and female chromosomes into a unique genetic combination. The possible number of these combinations is practically inexhaustible. We cannot therefore predict with any kind of accuracy what our offspring will be like. Their intelligence, temperament, talents, health, etc., all remain a mystery until they are born, and more precisely, until they reach maturity. This consideration is especially important with regard to the generation of human offspring. Because the source of man's dignity as well as his primary importance to society is his personhood, his ontological uniqueness as a self, the attempt to valorize him according to a type necessarily reduces, to a considerable extent, the possible number of genetic combinations and thus, by reducing the biological conditions, reduces the range of persons that can be conceived. And this, in turn, must progressively diminish the possibility of the unique contributions of a Socrates, St. Theresa of

Avila, Beethoven, Einstein, Churchill, Mother Teresa, etc.[23]

When it comes to the concrete particular entity, what we call the "individual," science is no better off — in fact, it is worse off — than philosophy; it cannot know the individual *as such* because the individual *as such* cannot be grasped conceptually; and since its control over nature depends upon its knowledge of things, it follows that its control over the individual must be as indirect and tentative as is its knowledge of it. Science operates from generalization and that is why its prodigious predictive power is limited to statistical frequencies and correlations. Scientific prediction is thus no more than highly sophisticated guessing; it calculates the probability of a given event occurring a given number of times according to a standard, say, one hundred *per cent*. As long as predictive success remains high, the failure of some of the entities in question to conform to the predication does not invalidate the hypothesis. But the significance of the failure rate depends upon the kind of entity under investigation, especially on whether it is human or subhuman. If human, then the failure of even only one out of every thousand or million or billion, or however vast a number you wish, is not necessarily to be written off as an insignificant anomaly. Because subhuman beings are not selves, the abstractive process by which scientific generalization reduces individuals having similar relevant properties to the same common denominator does not do violence to their nature. But human beings are selves; each is a center of the universe, his actions follow from a unique ontological interiority, and he is self-perfecting and self-determining. Consequently, the attempt to reduce his uniqueness, which is essentially and primarily ontological rather than psychological, to the common denominator of a type can radically violate the nature of the individual human being. If the generalization seeks simply to predict the frequency with which a certain biological type occurs, then obviously no violation takes place. But if the generalization ruled out of court as insignificant the individual *as such* (a dismissal encouraged perhaps because the individual *as such* cannot be absorbed intact into the generalization), then he could well suffer the violence of the Procrustean bed.

Intelligence, health, physical type, etc., in short all the things that supporters of eugenics have in mind when they call our attention to the types of men and women that they regard as desirable, are, in philosophical terms, "accidents;" the substance they do not know. Expressed in terms of the Aristotelian doctrine of substance and accident, they would know the accidents of their laboratory subjects directly, e.g., their intelligence or morphology, and their substances only indirectly, i.e., the concrete singular entity, "Adam." But the substance is the subject of the accidents: intelligence, let alone degree of intelligence, physical type, temperament, etc., do not exist by themselves but as modifications of the substance. It is after all this particular human being, "Adam," who has the intelligence. We say that the intellect knows when, accurately speaking, it it is the individual man who knows. [24]

Now here is the rub. Because, as accidents, intelligence, health, talent, etc., have no reality in themselves but derive it only insofar as they share in the existence of the substance — they are, in other words, ways of being — what is of primary importance is the substance, the concrete, singular entity. But since the substance cannot be known in its singularity, we must face the fact that we cannot know things, not, at any rate, with a direct conceptual knowledge, in their most important aspect. We can, to be sure, know the substance of Adam as "this particular human being." But this occurs through a combination of direct knowledge of his essence, *man* (a conceptual knowledge produced by the intellect's abstraction of the thing's intelligible form), which knowledge is then, by a reflexive action, returned to the concrete being of a specific type. Through intuition, a non-conceptual knowledge, we know that concrete singular as such and, *a fortiori*, know the concrete, singular human being, "Adam," in his singularity or uniqueness — which is to say in his selfhood, in the unique, unrepeatable person that he is.[25] But, although it is the highest, most important kind of knowledge, intuition *(intellectus)*, by the

very nature of its operation and object, does not lend itself
to conceptual formulation and thus eludes the embrace of
scientific methodology.

With regard to the scientific knowledge of subhuman beings, our inability to know the individual *as such*, although
admittedly a limitation, poses no important threat to their
dignity or to mankind for the simple reason that animals
are not persons, not unique centers of conscious,
autonomous being. That is why we regard the breeding of
animals for the production of offspring that embody the
ideal type as part of the natural order of things. Conversely, the value of a human being is precisely in his uniqueness as a subject. To breed men and women for an ideal
type, whether that be intelligence, talent, morphology, etc.,
is to invert the natural order by endeavoring to make the
substance serve the accidents. A stupid or sickly man is
every bit as dignified and valuable as an intelligent or
healthy one; each man and woman possesses a preeminent
dignity by virtue of an ontological interiority: each is a
person.

Here then is a second area where the Promethean aspiration overstretches itself, where Icarus flies too close to the
sun only to plummet into the sea to his destruction — the
inability of the human mind to know the individual *as such*
and thus the inability of science to grasp the human being
in his unique selfhood. In his masterful novel, *Dracula*,
Bram Stroker reveals insight into this point when he has
one of the characters observe:

> It looks like religious mania, and he will soon think
> that he himself is God. These infinitesmal distinctions
> between man and man are too paltry for an omnipo-
> tent being. How these madmen give themselves
> away! The real God taketh heed lest a sparrow fall;
> but the God created by human vanity sees no dif-
> ference between an eagle and a sparrow. Oh, if men
> only knew![26]

Add this limitation to that discussed above, namely, that
man creates only in an analogous sense, and you can see
the metaphysical basis for the destructive end to the Promethean creations in *Faust* and *Frankenstein*. The lesson of

these Promethean myths does not depend on the swift and cataclysmic occurrence of man's destruction. His destruction could as easily occur slowly and imperceptibly by a process of evisceration. Assume for the sake of argument that the laboratory reproduction of human beings in our own image and likeness — i.e., according to an ideal type — comes about. During and after its occurrence, the members of the human race might plausibly remain oblivious to the disaster. For, if breeding for an ideal type inevitably narrows the range of possible combinations of genes, thereby progressively delimiting the possible number of unique human beings coming into existence, there would most probably be no awareness of these lost possibilities. Those who did come into existence would, to be sure, be unique. But the totality of the contributions of these beings would be limited because it would be constricted by the possibilities contained in the ideal type. The reciprocal and overall influence of the widest number of unique beings is what the human species needs for its vitality and progress. Uniqueness of self, recall, is at the very heart of the dignity and value of the human person. And this uniqueness is, before he or she exists, unpredictable and, after that existence ends, irreplaceable. Thus the laboratory reproduction of human beings must produce an increasingly stereotypical man and woman. Although gradual, such a deterioration of creative, vital resources could, in the end, prove as destructive of the human race as a nuclear holocaust.

II
The Pivotal Ontological Consideration

Whether Pre-Christian, Christian, or Post-Christian, the Promethean myth proclaims the preeminent dignity of man in nature: man the knower, the seeker of knowledge, the very quest itself revealing his perception of himself as the inheritor of the universe. It is not simply man's right to know what the Promethean myth proclaims but, more fundamentally, his right to determine his own life and destiny. Only, the desire to know and the desire for self-determination are inextricably bound together. But bet-

ween the Christian and Post-Christian forms of Prometheanism stands a pivotal consideration which determines the meaning of man's dignity as a rational,
autonomous, creative agent. When you admit the existence
of God, you acknowledge the universe as a *creation,* as
something *given,*[27] because there is a "draughtsman," i.e.,
essences, intelligible structures, in things. (Although in the
order of discovery, the human mind proceeds in the op-
posite way: seeing that things are intelligible, that they embody essences, it is led to the conclusion that there must
exist a "draughtsman.") In the second part of his *Summa
Theologiae,* Thomas Aquinas represents essence such that
it is at once the sign of man's creaturehood and his imag-
ing of God. It seems to me that this representation is quite
pertinent to the task of reconciling human dignity and
human limitation:

> . . . law, being a rule and measure, can be in a person
> in two ways: in one way, as in him that rules and
> measures; in another way, as in that which is ruled
> and measured, since a thing is ruled and measured,
> in so far as it partakes of the rule or measure.
> Wherefore, since all things subject to Divine pro-
> vidence are ruled and measured by the eternal law
> . . . (,) it is evident that all things partake somewhat
> of the eternal law, in so far as, namely, from its being
> imprinted on them, they derive their respective in-
> clinations to their proper acts and ends. *Now among
> all others, the rational creature is subject to Divine pro-
> vidence in the most excellent way, in so far as it partakes
> of a share of providence, by being provident both for itself
> and for others. Whereof it has a share of the Eternal Reason,
> whereby it has a natural inclination to its proper act and
> end; and this participation of the eternal law in the rational
> creature is called the natural law.* [28] (Emphasis added)

If the natural law is the eternal law of God as the latter expresses itself in the being of creatures possessed of reason
and free will, it follows that, just because man is a creature,
he does not have perfect autonomy; he is not absolutely
self-determining. Although he directs his life by reason, he
nevertheless remains subject to the inclinations of his

essence. It is his essence ("blueprint") — what he has in common with all men *(unum in multis)* — rather than his unique selfhood which impels him to his final end of happiness in God. Even his intellect and will, the source of his preeminence in nature impressed upon him by the Creator determine his way of reasoning and choosing.[29]

If we accept the view that man is self-determining, but not absolutely so — and it seems to me that our experience confirms this view — then we have a rule and measure for reconciling man's preeminent dignity with this limitation which has its ground in what he essentially and really is. From a knowledge of man's essence — which is learned *experimentally (operatio sequitur esse*[30] — we learn two things: first, man has an essence and therefore is not undefined at the start of his life but is in fact specified so as to exist according to a predetermined intelligible structure. He does not create his own nature, but creatively actualizes the potentials as a man, and more precisely, as a unique embodiment of man. As a being of a specified type, he reveals himself as a being that is "ruled and measured:" second, we learn from the specificities of his essence that he has determinate finalities and exigencies, that he has a natural inclination to his "proper act and end."

Thus, although we cannot know a priori how we ought to behave in specific cases, say, of gene manipulation, what we have learned experimentally about man's essence indicates basic kinds of conduct that are immoral because contrary to the finalities of that essence. For example, treating men and women as mere means to an end, as mere objects of scientific research or social purpose: destroying human beings, whether in the blastula, embryo, or fetal stage, because they are growing deformed; producing men and women with varying degrees of intelligence (semimorons for menial work, e.g.,) or with physiological anomalies to increase dexterity in the performance of certain specialized tasks, such as with abnormally short legs attached to a normal sized torso with stooped shoulders for working in mines or other troglodytic ventures.

In itself the conclusion that we are to base our decisions concerning the genetic manipulation of mankind on the exigencies and finalities of our essence is anticlimactic. As a statement of the ontological basis of ethics it is unexceptionable. But we have seen that the Promethean challenge runs deeper than the search for moral norms. It arises out of the frustration of the creature who would share the infinite knowledge and power of God. Now, in addition to supplying the basis for moral conduct, the pivotal ontological consideration plumbs the depths of the Promethean challenge and points the way to the reconciliation of man's creaturehood with his desire to be like God.

To be at once "that which is ruled and measured" and a being "who rules and measures" generates frustration only when knowledge is subordinated to power. The subordination may well reflect the ancient confusion of knowledge with magic, but in the modern age knowledge and power surge together spontaneously from the application of the univocal conception of knowing to science. For its advances in knowledge, science relies upon hypothesis and prediction, a methodology that has proved itself to be prodigiously successful. So tightly does this methodology bind together knowing and the exercise of power over nature that one can easily be led to affirm Bacon's dictum, "Knowledge is power." And when knowledge is conceived univocally and human knowing is thus enshrined as the paradigm of knowing, then the subordination of knowledge to power is complete. For, as argued above, if the criterion of knowledge is that which is clear and distinct (to the intellect of man), then it is inevitable that a method which vindicates knowledge by increasing his control over nature will become the standard of knowledge. Thus the method of hypothesis and prediction can easily be reinterpreted to mean "knowledge is manipulation." John Dewey, for example, who could not have been more emphatic in his approval of the dictum, "Knowledge is power," argued that we can properly say that we know a thing only to the extent that we can bend it to our will.[31]

Moreover, the intimate connection in scientific methodology between knowing and the exercise of power cannot help but arouse charges of obscurantism against those who argue that the laboratory reproduction of human beings ought not to be pursued. After all, does not the curtailment of scientific research in any given area impose constraints on the pursuit of knowledge and thereby obstruct human progress?

To see the proper connection between knowledge and power, a brief analysis of knowledge is in order. The analysis requires, however, a change in terminology. Because power is a species of action, the more accurate juxtaposition is that between knowledge and action rather than between knowledge and power. Because what is true of the genus must be true of the species, what is true of action must accordingly be true of power. What will emerge from the analysis of knowledge is that no opposition exists between knowledge and action because knowing is the most perfect form of action.

To illustrate this point, let us ask ourselves what a perfect act is. Any act in which an agent acts upon a being outside himself is imperfect in this sense, that the former's activity is not for himself but for the other. For example, the surgeon operates on the patient to improve the latter's health rather than to benefit himself. Of course, the surgeon benefits, but only indirectly: the practice of surgery improves his skills and most likely he gets paid for his services. Whatever the surgeon's personal motives for operating on the patient, the fact remains that the art of surgery derives its rationale from the goal of healing; it exists for the benefit of the sick. Thus the surgeon, *as surgeon,* is dependent on the sick, for if no one were sick, there would be no need for surgery.[32] In contrast, an act which by its very nature directly benefits the agent is a perfect act and is called *immanent* because its activity is, in the end, ontological, for it is the activity of a being that exists for its own sake rather than for an other.[33]

Knowing is the prime example of immanent activity. That knowing is primarily understanding *(intellectus)* as opposed to discursive *(ratio)* reveals itself in a consideration of the goal of all thinking that may be called "problem solving" — understanding. This kind of thinking is discursive because in doing it we move from what we know to a knowledge of what was previously unknown. Thus it is correct to say that discursive thinking is imperfect knowledge because perplexity, ignorance and doubt are its muses. Were we free from these states of mind, we should have no need for this kind of thinking. Because its rationale is understanding, discursive thinking is a transitive activity and is therefore imperfect activity. This is not, however, to suggest that discursive thinking occurs independently of understanding at any given moment. For it is quite clear that, as we reason our way from A to B, we simultaneously *understand* the terms of the reasoning. Nevertheless, the discursive process betrays our imperfection as intellectual substances, for it signals that we are only "on the way" to understanding. Once we solve the problem, we have arrived at the state of intellection, i.e., understanding; there we have the *raison d'etre* for discursive thinking and there our intellectual labors come to rest. If discursive thinking is for the sake of understanding, understanding is for the sake of nothing else; as an immanent act, it is a perfect act. To say that understanding is for its own sake is to speak of understanding *as such*. Understanding arrived at as successive stages in problem solving facilitates the solution of further problems and is assigned an instrumental value. But in science, philosophy, literature, and art — which is to say in higher reaches of human thought — the goal is understanding and nothing more.

The pursuit of understanding for its own sake permits man to transcend the tension between his preeminence and creaturehood by establishing the priority between knowledge and power. In this accomplishment is vindicated the finest impulse expressed in the Promethean Myth, for it reconciles man's desire to share the infinite power and knowledge of God — to be a being "who rules and measures" — with assertion that there are some things which he not only cannot achieve but which he ought not to attempt — a reminder that he is also "that which is ruled and measured."

It is knowledge for the sake of understanding which confers on man genuine mastery over things. This can be certified by a consideration of our dealings with the material world. As we had occasion to observe earlier, a fundamental indication that we are creators only in an analogous sense is that our creativity is limited by the predeterminations of preexistent matter. Despite our prodigious technological achievements, our mastery over matter remains tenuous; we never master the material world completely: we fell trees and and crush rock to build our structures; but wood rots and concrete crumbles. We transform fossils into fuel, but the pollution of our atmosphere is a serious side-effect. In its inner structure matter is irreducible and accordingly successfully resists our attempts at total domination.[34]

In knowing, on the contrary, we master things completely. Knowing is a becoming of the thing by the knower.[35] Knowing consists in the knowing subject apprehending the essential structure of the thing known. Because knowing is a becoming, the knowing subject thus masters the thing in its innermost being. Intellect therefore more perfectly masters its object than does will, for the latter is confined to a purely external relation to things.[36] Again, because knowing is a becoming of the other *as other*, it reveals itself as the primary way in which it is true to say that man is in God's image and likeness. Becoming the other *as other*, man overcomes the limitations of his finite being insofar as he can thereby become all other things, and all the while retain his unique selfhood: it is always *I*, the unique self-aware subject that I am, who knows. Thus the individual man, who is a unique center of the universe, can, through knowing, unify the fragmentation and plurality of the universe within himself: as a knower, man is *virtually* infinite.[37]

We are now in a position to address the charge, alluded to above, that the proscription of specific areas of scientific research obstructs human progress. Consider the difference between "problem" and a "mystery." A problem lends itself to a solution; all that is required is that the pieces of the puzzle be fitted together, a feat that very often depends on the discovery of new data. A mystery, on the other hand, has no solution; the discovery of new data is irrelevant. Instead, we penetrate ever more deeply into the reality of it. Thus the progress of knowing, *as understanding,* is genuine progress. The advances made in problem-solving, the *modus operandi* of the sciences, are more correctly termed *advance by overthrow and replacement* than *progress,* for there is often no continuity in the change from one scientific view to its replacement.[38] The discovery of fresh data often results in the falsification and abandonment of long standing theories. But knowing, as understanding, is genuine progress because as our understanding of reality deepens, we witness the marriage of continuity and change. Continuity because it is one and the same reality our intellect continues to penetrate, the nature of man, say, or beauty, without the addition of new data; change because our knowledge of reality thereby deepens.

The immanent nature of knowing reveals another facet of the preeminent dignity of man. Because knowing is an immanent act, it is, we have seen, a self-perfecting act: the act is its own justification; it is identical with its goal. Now a being capable of a self-perfecting act is a being that is itself self-perfecting and is accordingly a being that exists for itself. Conversely, where knowing is subordinated to power, knowledge can claim only an instrumental value, for its value is contingent upon its capacity to contribute to the manipulation of its object. Thus to seek the rationale for knowing entirely or even primarily in problem-solving is to assign a purely or primarily instrumental value to knowing. But this can only result in the eclipse of the self-perfecting nature of knowing. Where transitive rather than immanent activity is adorned with pride of place, it is inevitable that man descend from the status of a self-perfecting being who exists in some important sense for his own sake, as an end in himself — the human species, for example — a mere means to an end. The valorization of knowing purely or primarily in terms of problem-solving reduces itself, we have seen, to the principle, "Knowledge is power." The affirmation of this principle cannot help but unleash a demiurgical force before which everything — politics, morals, art, science and philosophy, even man himself — must submit to the imperatives of power.[39] In the specific area of scientific endeavor that falls into the category of the biological revolution, this reduction of knowledge to power will play out no differently: the project of improving the human species by laboratory reproduction and various forms of genetic engineering will suffer not only from the previously discussed liabilities inherent in creaturely power and knowledge but also from the instrumentalist error of valorizing man entirely or primarily in terms of his usefulness. Besides debasing man who is a being "who is a rule and measure" as well as a being "which is ruled and measured," it rivets the Promethean impulses to the horizontal plane, thereby preventing any transcendence of the tension between creaturehood and the desire for the Absolute.

We come now full circle to our earlier discussion of the deification of man through the misconception of knowledge as a univocal notion. The validity of the scientific methodology of hypothesis and predication depends on the analogous notion of knowledge with God as the primary analogate, on the divine knowing as the paradigm of knowing. As a perfectly immanent act, knowing is the most perfect form of action. The first conclusion to be drawn from this is that ultimately no opposition exists between knowing and action; indeed, knowing is the most intense and powerful form of action.[40] The second is that since God is the absolutely perfect being, His action must be absolutely free of dependence on others and absolutely for Himself alone; and since knowing, as understanding, knowing for its own sake, is the most perfect form of action because it is a perfectly immanent act, it follows that knowing is the Divine action; and since He is absolutely self-sufficient and independent, the object of His knowledge must be Himself alone. Thus not only must God know all things, possible and actual, by knowing Himself, the first of all actions, i.e., the fiat by which the universe came into being, must have been the Divine self-knowledge. In knowing himself, therefore, God possesses the unity and fullness of being. In contrast, man, the creature, is a diminished intellectual substance who must accordingly rely upon things outside himself for his knowledge. In knowing them, he overcomes his own limitations as well as reunifying the fragmented, diverse beings that comprise the created universe within himself.[41] Thus whereas God and His knowledge are absolutely unified from start to finish, so to speak, man must work his way from plurality to unity, and he does this preeminently through knowing.

Discursive knowing, or problem-solving, characterizes the human situation: owing to man's limitation as an enfleshed knower caught up in time and materiality, it is a necessary means to the goal of understanding; in the material world, transitive action is the means to immanent action, work the means to leisure, problem-solving and struggle the means to contemplation. Within this framework, man enjoys his foretaste of identification with the Absolute and Infinite in this life. As Aristotle observed, it is in contemplation that we are most like the divine.[42] Here then knowledge and power, creaturehood and the yearning to be like God are reconciled in the perfect action that is knowing.

Conclusion
I said at the outset of this presentation that the biological revolution in itself poses no threat to mankind and that if Christian, rather than post-Christian, Prometheanism were the driving force behind it, the Promethean *elan* would be channeled so as to produce an improvement in the human species as genuine as it would be spectacular. Consider, for example, the prospect of genetic engineering, and specifically "gene therapy." Although we are now nowhere near the day when we shall be able to replace or repair dysfunctional genes, it remains nevertheless a goal worthy of our best efforts. From the vantage point of what I have called "the pivotal ontological consideration," we have, through experiential knowledge, an inderstanding of our human nature — that by which we are "ruled and measured" — which nature is the blueprint according to which we could use gene therapy to eliminate neuro-psychological impediments to the full expression of its potentials. Think of what it would mean to eliminate, once

and for all, from the human race the scourge of Downs Syndrome! Thus that by which we are "ruled and measured" supplies us with an answer to Jonathan Glover's question, "What Sort of People Should There Be?" Man's nature, or essence, is the Divine proclamation of what he is and can be. Because we are also beings who "rule and measure," our challenge is to use our reason, freedom, and creativity to fulfill the potentials of our nature.

I have argued that to be that which is "ruled and measured" is to be a creature and that the latter condition determines not only *what we ought not to do* but also *what we cannot do.* The lesson of the Promethean Myth is that to attempt them is to destroy oneself. But I have further argued that the acknowledgement of these creaturely limitations does not condemn us to the unrelievable frustration of desiring to be like God and yet never being able to fulfill that desire. That is the result of the rebellion against God, which rebellion implies the absurdity of denying man's intrinsic ontological insufficiency and dependency. On the contrary, because we cannot create in the absolute sense and because we ought not to try to create human beings as if we were breeding animals, it does not follow that we must abandon our attempts to emulate the infinitude of God, that we thus voluntarily erect barriers to human progress. For on many levels our laboratory research will carry us forward to ever fuller realizations of man's essence. But, at all events, the integrity of his essence should fill us with the wonder of God's creation and through the contemplation of his works raise us to higher and higher levels of being. Let us say that rather than leading us to derogate man's striving for increasing power over his existence, the acknowledgement of knowing as the most perfect form of action enables us to see that man's greatest power, that in which he most emulates God, is through the contemplative activity of knowing for the sake of understanding. Providing us with a vertical ascent, the latter uplifts the purely horizontal advance of transitive activities, in this case, the problem-solving activity and predictive goals of science, so that our biological researches will always be accompanied by an increasingly transcendent view of man and his relation to nature and God. Christian Prometheanism leads therefore to authentic progress, while post-Christian Prometheanism, in its rivalry of God, generated nothing more than the illusion of progress. Goethe wrote Part II of *Faust* in the reflective wisdom of old age. In the past he describes Wagner's successful generation of human life in a flask. In contrast to Wagner's joy upon seeing the homunculus, Goethe assigns Mephistopheles the task of a rather more sober observation:

He who lives long a host of things will know,
The world affords him nothing new to see.
Much have I seen, in wandering to and fro,
Including crystallized humanity.[44]

Perhaps it would be well to mount these words in all laboratories and studies where the biological revolution is seen to hold the hope of the future.

Footnotes

1. Jonathan Glover, *What Sort of People Should There Be?* (Harmondsworth, Middlesex, England: Penguin Books Ltd., 1984)
2. Jeremy Rifkin, *Algeny* (Harmondsworth, Middlesex, England: Penguin Books Ltd., 1984), Part One.
3. Glover, pp. 130 ff.
4. James Schall, S.J., *The Politics of Heaven and Hell* (Lanham, Maryland: The University Press of America, 1984), p. 141; see also Ch VIII.
5. Schall, Ch VI.
6. David Ketterer, *Frankenstein's Creation: the book, the monster, and human reality* (Victoria, B.C.: University of Victoria, 1979), 19-20
7. Johann Wolfgang Goethe, *Faust*. tr. by Carlyle I. MacIntyre (Norfolk: New Directions, 1941), (2 vols.) Vol. I, part I, p. 35.
8. Bettina Knapp, *The Prometheus Syndrome* (Troy, New York: The Whitston Publishing Co., 1970), pp. 91-2.
9. Goethe, *Faust*, tr. by Philip Wayne (Baltimore: Penguin Books, 1959) (2 vols.), Vol. 2, Part II, pp. 91-2.
10. Mary Wollstonecraft Shelley, *Frankenstein or the Modern Prometheus* (New York: The Heritage Press, no date)
11. Knapp, ch. on Albertus Magnus.
12. Henri de Lubac, S.J., *The Drama of Atheist Humanism*, tr. by Edith M. Riley (London: Sheed & Ward, 1949), p.97
13. See, e.g., Pope John Paul II *Redemptor Hominis*, #14
14. Carl Grabo, *Prometheus Unbound: An Interpretation*. (Chapel Hill: The University of North Carolina Press, 1935). pp. 14-15 and esp. 185; Percy Bysshe Shelley, *Prometheus Unbound*, III, iv (8-130); IV, (554-78)
15. Ludwig Feuerbach, *The Essence of Christianity*, tr. by George Elliot (New York: Harper & Row, 1957), pp. 2-3, 38-39; but esp. 40-41 & 153.
16. Feuerbach, p. 91
17. Feuerbach, pp. 152-3
18. Fyodor Dostoyevsky, *The Possessed*, tr. by Constance Garnett (New York: Dell Publishing Co. Inc., 1961), Pt. III, Ch 6, pp. 630-41
19. Quoted in Ketterer, pp.11
20. Herbert Butterfield, *The Origins of Modern Science* (New York: The MacMillan Company, 1960) Ch VIII, esp. pp. 151 ff.
21. Goethe, *Faust*, MacIntyre transl., Vol. I, Part I, p. 35
22. Jacques Maritain, *St. Thomas Aquinas*. Newly transl. & revised by Joseph W. Evans and Peter O'Reilly (New York: The World Publishing Co., 1962), pp. 91-92; see also Knapp, p. 156.
23. "The primary role of sex is more subtle than straightforward reproduction: it is the creation of genetic diversity among offspring. An organism that reproduces without sex, say by hatching unfertilized eggs, can replicate itself exactly, gene by gene, without wasting time on courtship. But if all the offspring are identical, they are less likely as a group to withstand important changes in the environment. Suppose that a disease sweeping through the area kills all the individuals with the mother's hereditary makeup. If the mother has reproduced in a nonsexual manner, she and all of her offspring would perish. But if she had mated with a male bearing disease-resistant genes, at least some of her offspring would survive. Also surviving would be the tendency to reproduce sexually; sex itself can be said to be favored by natural selection. Sex is slower than nonsex, but it provides a balanced array of genetic combinations to present to the

world. It spreads the hereditary investment, including all the time and energy that go into reproduction, in a way that copes more consistently with harsh and constantly changing environments. Most biologists agree that adaptability, the general ability to adapt, is just as important as adaptiveness, the actual set of responses made by organisms to the environemnt that keeps them alive and allows them to reproduce. This long-term property is what has given sex an edge through eons of evolution and fixed it in the biology of most kinds of organisms." C. Lumsden and E. Wilson, *Promethean Fire* (Cambridge, Mass:Harvard University Press, 1979), p. 28

24. Raymond Dennehy, *Reason and Dignity* (Washington, D.C.: University Press of America, 1981), pp. 43-48.
25. Pierre Rousselot, *The Intellectualism of St. Thomas.* Trans by Father James E. O'Mahoney (New York: Sheed & Ward, Inc., 1935), pp. 97-98. See also Jacques Maritain, *Existence and the Existent.* Tr. by Lewis Galantiere and Gerald B. Phelan (Garden City, New York: Doubleday & Company, Inc., 1956), pp. 81-87.
26. Bram Stoker, *Dracula* (Garden City, New York: Garden City Books, no date), p.95
27. Raymond Dennehy, "The Social Encyclicals: What Has Heaven to Do with Earth?" *Faith and Reason* VIII (Fall, 1982) 232-246, p. 234
28. Thomas Aquinas, *Summa Theologiae* I-II, 91, 2 in *Basic Writings of Saint Thomas Aquinas.* Edited by Anton C. Pegis (New York: Random House, 1945) (2 vols), Vol. II, pp. 749-750
29. Thomas Aquinas, *Summa Theologiae,* I, 18, a.'s 1-3.
30. *Summa Theologiae,* I, 89, a.1
31. John Dewey, *Reconstruction in Philosophy* (1948; rpt. Boston: Beacon Press, 1957), Ch III, esp. pp. 114-115.
32. Aristotle, *Metaphysics,* IX, Ch 8, 1050a 24-1050b
33. Rousselot, pp. 25-26
34. *Reason and Dignity,* pp.46-50
35. *Reason and Dignity,* p. 48
36. *Summa Theologiae* I, 76, a.5, ad.4
37. Maritain, *Preface to Metaphysics* (New York: Books For Libraries, 1979), pp. 2-5. For the several positions on the significance of scientific advance see Thomas S. Kuhn, *The Structure of Scientific Revolutions* 2nd ed. (Chicago: University of Chicago Press, 1975), Paul Feyerabend, *Against Method* (London: Humanities Press, 1975), and W.H. Newton-Smith, *The Rationality of Science* (London: Routledge and Kegan Paul, 1981.).
38. Dennehy, "Education, Vocationalism, and Democracy," *Thought* LVII (June 1982) 182-195, pp. 191-194.
39. Rousselot, p. 24
40. Aquinas, *Contra Gentiles,* Ch 11; Rousselot, pp. 8-9- & 24
41. Aristotle, *Nicomachean Ethics,* X, Ch 8, 1179a 11-31
42. *Faust,* tr. by Philip Wayne, Part II, Vol. II, p. 100

II. A CHRISTIAN ETHICS OF LIMITING MEDICAL TREATMENT: GUIDANCE FOR PATIENTS, PROXY DECISION MAKERS, AND COUNSELORS
by Germain Grisez

A. Presuppositions

Unless the context indicates otherwise, "medical treatment" will be used here in a wide sense, to include all forms of treatment and care, including ordinary nursing care, carried out under a physician's direction to promote health or maintain life.

Life is a basic human good; much we do has no purpose but to serve it. Human life also is sacred; it is God's great gift. Faith makes clear the value of bodily life: Sin leads to death; reconciliation with God leads to bodily resurrection.

People naturally cherish life. But despite this natural inclination, one can neglect health problems due to sluggishness, live unhygienically due to lack of self-control, or fail to get needed treatment due to excessive fear. Thus, there is a general, affirmative moral responsibility to overcome laziness, self-indulgence, and cowardice, and to seek needed treatment.

Those who can make decisions for themselves should not try to evade their personal responsibility. Like every other decision in life, decisions about medical treatment should take into account one's commitments and other duties, and should be adapted to one's unique personality, gifts, and limitations. Others cannot take all these factors into account as well as patients themselves can.

For any noncompetent person, some competent person must make decisions about many matters, including medical treatment. I call such decisions "proxy decisions." The proxy decision maker should try to make the very decisions the patient would make, assuming the patient were morally upright and competent.

Hospital administrators, physicians, and others with technical expertise can provide helpful information to clarify options worth considering. But they are not suitable proxies for noncompetent patients. A good proxy must know the patient intimately and have the whole of the patient's personal interests at heart. But interests of professionals are likely to conflict with some of a patient's legitimate personal interests. If a noncompetent patient is a member of a good, Christian family, its usual way of making decisions generally will be the best way to reach proxy decisons about treatment.

The goodness of human life and God's lordship over it have led all faithful Jews and Christians to live by an absolute moral norm: Without God's clear authorization, one may never deliberately kill a human being. It was believed that God authorized capital punishment, some killing in war, and so on. But in the matters dealt with here, there is no exception to the divine command: You shall not kill.

B. What will not be considered here

Questions about limiting medical treatment often are important and difficult, and so decisions often are disputed. One function of the law is to prevent or settle dispute. So discussions about limiting treatment often concern what the law ought to be. I have dealt with this elsewhere; here I will be concerned only with what the moral truth is.

Among the presuppositions stated above is the Jewish and Christian norm which forbids deliberately killing the innocent. Many today reject this moral absolute, and say that in conflict situations, one must choose the so-called lesser evil. This view will be ignored here, for I have shown elsewhere that it is both rationally indefensible and incompatible with Catholic faith.

Nor will I consider here questions about the responsibilities of physicians, nurses, and so on. The ethics of the patient's or proxy's role is more basic; they should be the principal decision makers. Acting as servants, health-care professionals need only fulfill their trust and avoid doing anything wrong. Patients and proxies must try to discern what is right, considering everything, including personal factors only they can assess.

Sometimes a decision — e.g., whether or not to switch off a respirator — turns on whether the body is a corpse or a living person. However, I have treated the question of the definition of death elsewhere and will not treat it here. Thus, what follows assumes that there is still a living patient.

Finally, ethical reflection tries to clarify the moral truth to which decisions should conform; it does not try to judge hearts. Hence, what follows should not be read as a moral condemnation of people who have acted, presumably in good faith, according to norms which I will criticize.

C. What will be considered here

Sometimes people choose to limit the medical treatment they will receive. The limitation might extend to refusal of all treatment, or stop short of that. Bad reasons for such choices to limit will be considered in section D. People sometimes also have bad reasons, to be considered in section E, for choosing to continue or seek additional treatment.

Under certain conditions, to be considered in section F, people ought to limit medical treatment for themselves. Under other conditions, to be considered in section G, people are not obliged to limit medical treatment they will receive, but may rightly do so.

The moral norms of proxy judgments on behalf of non-competent patients are the norms of the corresponding judgments people make on their own behalf. But applying these norms in proxy judgments involves special difficulties, to be clarified in section H.

Finally, counselors try to help both competent persons and proxies for others to make sound decisions. Besides the norms decision makers themselves should follow, counselors should shape their own activity by special norms, to be considered in section I.

D. Bad reasons for limiting medical treatment

It is presupposed here that the deliberate killing of the innocent is always wrong. Deliberate suicide is a kind of deliberate killing. So it is always wrong. A choice to limit medical treatment can be a choice of a way of committing suicide. If it is, that is always a bad reason to limit treatment.

To apply this norm, one must understand clearly when a choice to limit medical treatment is the choice of a method of committing suicide. Not every action which brings about one's death is a case of committing suicide. A suicidal action can be performed — e.g., by a severely depressed person — without a free choice. In such cases, the self-killing is not deliberate.

Moreover, one can deliberately do something which leads to one's death without deliberately killing oneself. One can freely accept death without committing suicide. Suicide is the direct killing of oneself. What does that mean?

Whenever one acts deliberately, one has confronted two or more options for acting, considered the pros and cons of each one, and settled the indeterminacy of the situation by making a free choice. The open options about which one deliberates are proposals, very like motions on the floor of a deliberative body. Proposals point to opportunities to achieve some good or avoid something bad, and include a plan for bringing about the desired outcome. In adopting a proposal by one's free choice, one determines oneself to live by the values it promises and to execute its plan.

A person who deliberately commits suicide considers continued life somehow bad — e.g., more painful than pleasant. The proposal to kill oneself comes to mind, with at least some idea of how one might do it. But a counterproposal, to continue living, also comes to mind. The moral act of suicide begins with the adoption of the proposal — i.e., with the choice — to kill oneself. The carrying out of that proposal's plan is the direct killing of oneself.

Obviously, one need not formulate a suicidal proposal in terms of killing oneself. One might say to oneself something equivalent in meaning: "I could end it all." Or one might specify the deadly means to be used: "I could take all these sleeping pills at once." The plan to bring about one's death also can be by omission: "I could refuse to accept this treatment." And if it were pointed out to the person who has chosen suicide, "By refusing this treatment, you will be killing yourself," the honest reply would be: "That is exactly what I propose to do."

The carrying out of a plan of action often has important effects which one foresees during deliberation but which are no part of the proposal one adopts. The person who chooses suicide, for example, may foresee that others will be saddened, not desire that, but accept it as an unwanted side effect.

One's death itself can be a foreseen side effect of carrying out a plan not chosen for that reason. Jesus' plan was to carry on his work despite opposition. He foresaw and freely accepted death as a side effect of going up to Jerusalem. He did not directly kill himself. Similarly, a person who rejects burdensome treatment may foresee and freely accept death without adopting a suicidal proposal. Accepting death to avoid burdensome treatment may or may not be morally upright, but it is not direct killing of oneself.

Thus, not everyone who limits needed treatment, knowing that death will result, deliberately commits suicide. But one who does not seek or who terminates needed treatment in executing a plan to hasten death does deliberately commit suicide. Since such deliberate killing is always wrong, no ulterior reason for wishing to be dead can justify it. However, its wrongness can be mitigated by an ulterior reason, such as the desire not to be a burden to others.

The same outward behavior can carry out a choice to commit suicide by limiting treatment, or a nonsuicidal choice to avoid its burdens by limiting it, knowing that death will result. If the outward behavior and its results are exactly the same, why is the suicidal choice always morally evil and the nonsuicidal choice sometimes morally good? Because morality mainly concerns the heart — i.e., choices and other interior acts which accompany them. In adopting a proposal to kill oneself, one sets one's heart against the value of human life and against God, the Lord of life. In adopting a proposal to avoid the burdens of treatment by limiting it, knowing that death will result, one may or may not be upright in other respects, but one does not set one's heart against the value of life, and so need not offend God.

Probably many who commit suicide by limiting treatment think: There is nothing left for me to live for. But this reason also can motivate people who do not directly kill themselves. It is always a bad reason, because it is always false. Everyone who can make choices and communicate them to others has something to live for.

A person who can make and communicate choices can do other things. True, such a person can be virtually certain that the future holds more suffering than enjoyment. Yet this situation offers an opportunity to confront suffering courageously — to live with genuine dignity while dying. That itself is something to do, and since doing it is not easy, it is not only upright but noble.

Christians, moreover, should recognize that suffering is part of the way of the Lord Jesus, which they are called to follow through its bitter end in this world to the joy of heaven. God has prepared a life of good deeds for each of us to live, for the praise of his glory. As long as we can make choices, we have unfinished work. We are called to be faithful servants, and a faithful servant does not quit before quitting time. Moreover, the Christian must not only receive God's gifts and thank him for them, but share them with others. By meekly accepting suffering and by manifesting confident hope, the dying Christian, strengthened by the sacraments, engages in a very important apostolate: to remind others, especially those forgetful of life's meaning, of the Gospel's basic message: Repent, the kingdom of God is at hand.

E. Bad reasons for not limiting medical treatment

As in all else, moderation is needed in respect to medical treatment. Just as there are some inherently bad reasons for limiting treatment, there are some inherently bad reasons for seeking or continuing it.

One of these bad reasons often is expressed somewhat as follows: Since it is my body, and since I can afford it (or have insurance to cover the costs), nothing should be spared in treatment. Everything possible must be done.

This reason ignores the scarcity of medical facilities and services, and demands the use of unlimited resources to satisfy one person's desires. But the goods of nature and fruits of human effort used in medical treatment are gifts of God. Like all his gifts, they are to benefit all humankind, not simply the wealthy. Therefore, even if one's needs are genuine, at some point their satisfaction ought to be limited to allow some satisfaction of others' needs. But selfish reasoning simply disregards others' needs. That is unfair; it violates the Golden Rule.

In the United States and some other wealthy nations, a small fraction of the world's people want and get too much medical treatment. Their level of demand, the monopolisitc structure of medical services, and other factors combine to yield exorbitant incomes for some health-care professionals and to make medical, hospital, and laboratory bills spiral out of control. Meanwhile, the needs of the very poor for treatment receive scant attention.

Another bad reason for immoderately seeking and continuing medical treatment is pride, which leads some to refuse to accept death. This refusal often reinforces greed for treatment, but sometimes stands alone as a reason for making unjustifiable demands for it. One can sympathize with those who proudly refuse to accept death, for it is horrible; no realistic and honest person sees anything good in death, considered in itself. But it is inevitable, and so fully reasonable people adjust to it. Moreover, while God did not make death, he permits Adam's children to suffer death as a deserved punishment for sin, and so faithful Christians accept inevitable death with meekness and in a penitential spirit.

A third bad reason for immoderate demands for treatment is cowardice in the face of suffering and death. Again, one can sympathize with the anxiety of anyone afflicted with a serious injury or illness. However, this anxiety does not excuse a quest for false reassurance through excessive treatment. Moreover, faithful Christians should hope so confidently for everlasting life that they can rather easily let go of this mortal life, so that by dying in Christ they may rise to glory with him.

F. Reasons which require one to limit medical treatment

There can be conditions which not only justify one in

limiting medical treatment but require one to do so.

First, sometimes physicians and others propose forms of treatment which cannot be accepted without formal or unjustifiable material cooperation in moral evils. For example, certain forms of sex therapy involve masturbation, fornication, or adultery.

Second, sometimes accepting or continuing certain forms of treatment will interfere with fulfillment of other responsibilities. For example, otherwise acceptable levels of sedation might interfere with a particular patient's duty to make a last will or receive the sacrament of penance. Again, treatment, in a hospital which forbids visits by children might interfere with a dying mother's responsibility to instruct her children so that they will accept her death in the light of faith.

Third, sometimes particular patients who can profit little from beginning or continuing medical treatment encounter the clear limit of their fair share of available facilities and services. The most obvious example is a disaster situation, in which many survivors will have a good chance of recovery if they are cared for promptly. Those likely to die no matter what is done for them cannot fairly claim more than quick palliative care, if more extensive treatment for them would prevent adequate treatment for those with better chances. Fairness similarly requires indirect limits on treatment, through reasonable limits on public payments and insurace coverages.

Must one refuse pain-relieving drugs if an adequate dosage will certainly block the use of reason, probably induce addiction, and possibly hasten death? Not necessarily. If patients are not prevented from fulfilling their responsibilities, they need not refuse adequate pain relief because it blocks their use of reason. Patients with a prospect of recovery normally are not offered pain-relieving drugs in dosages which might addict or kill them; if inappropriate therapy is offered, it should be rejected. Dying patients usually will not be severely harmed if they become addicted to drugs used in dosages adequate to relieve their pain; hence, they may take the drugs and need not be concerned about becoming addicted to them. And while it is wrong for dying patients to hasten death deliberately, they need not refuse drugs adequate to relieve their pain and chosen for that purpose, even if they foresee side effects which will surely shorten life.

G. Factors which do not require but can justify limiting treatment

Several factors, which do not require upright persons to refuse or discontinue medical treatment, nevertheless can be good reasons to limit it. Since these factors ground negative judgments regarding treatment, they necessarily involve its bad features and effects. These negative aspects can be grouped in six categories.

First, medical treatment can be too costly. "Cost" can mean the use of scarce resources of individuals or families, of particular treatment systems, or of societies at large. At each level, choices must be made, and at some point prior to that at which it becomes clearly unfair to others to accept or continue treatment, the cost factor can make it reasonable to limit it.

Second, some medical treatment can be too damaging to one's bodily self and functioning. For example, a woman who hopes to have a child might not consent to a recommended hysterectomy. Again, a cancer patient might refuse chemotherapy because of its side effects on various bodily functions.

Third, medical treatment can be too painful. Courageous patients patiently accept some pain, but reasonably draw a line.

Fourth, medical treatment can be too repugnant psychologically — e.g., too embarrassing or too annoying. Upright patients generally overcome their repugnance, but, again, there are limits. For instance, an elderly patient with many health problems might become annoyed with the routine of hospital life and prefer simpler though less adequate care elsewhere.

Fifth, medical treatment can be too restrictive on a patient's physical liberty and preferred outward behavior. For example, someone given a year to live, with regular medical treatment and hospitalization, might prefer to take a trip, although doing so is incompatible with prescribed treatment.

Sixth, medical treatment can have too great an impact on a patient's inner life and activity. For example, patients who prefer to be alert and clear headed might refuse treatments which interfere with mental functions.

These six categories of negative aspects of treatment do not include three categories often mentioned: too burdensome, too risky, and useless.

Burdensomeness is not an additional category alongside the six mentioned, but the genus of which they are species. Thus, cost is one sort of burdensomeness, painfulness another, and so on. Risk is some probability that a treatment will lead to some great burden. Thus, riskiness is always reducible to one or more of the six categories mentioned.

Uselessness also is omited. Treatment is called "useless" either in a loose or in a strict sense. Treatment is called "useless" in a loose sense when its prospective benefits are considered insignificant in comparison with its great burdens. Treatment is called "useless" in a strict sense when what in other circumstances would be useful treatment becomes utterly pointless — a sheer waste of scarce resources. For example, if a patient is just as likely to die soon with or without major surgery, which meanwhile will do nothing to improve the patient's functioning or comfort, then for that patient the surgery is not truly treatment, and the materials, facilities, and services it involves are wasted. Hence, uselessness strictly so-called not only justifies but demands that efforts at treatment be terminated just insofar as they are useless. Of course, other sorts of treatment will remain appropriate.

Each of the six species of burdens includes the qualifier "too" — "too costly," "too painful," and so on — which signifies excess. Excess is a matter of proportion, and so all these reasons which justify limiting treatment raise questions of due proportion. The proportion is between negative aspects involved in or consequent on the treatment itself, and the benefits it offers the patient — prolonged life, improved health, preserved or restored function-g, lessened discomfort, and so forth. Potentially bad features always present in treatment become reasons which justify limiting it when prospective benefits are judged insufficient to make using the means worthwhile. How does one rightly make such a judgment?

In one of two ways, I think. The first — and most common where life is not at stake — is a conscientious discernment, by which all one's duties are taken into account. The second, more common in extreme situations, is by recognition that one has fulfilled the general, affirmative responsibility to seek or accept needed treatment, that no other responsibility calls one to go on with it, and that one simply has no desire to do so.

The judgment by conscientious discernment to limit medical treatment is put into proper perspective by noticing that upright persons regard virtually everything they do in life as the fulfillment of one responsibility or another. Good Christians try to do everything in the name of the Lord Jesus; through him, their whole lives become a gift of thanks to the Father. In their unique gifts and opportunities for service, good Christians find their personal vocations, and so organize their entire lives by faith in Christ, to do their part in the common enterprise of building up his body, the Church.

And so sleeping and rising, cleaning up and dressing, praying and working, eating and drinking, playing and shopping, and getting medical treatment — all fulfill affirmative responsibilities, which are parts of a unified life plan, a Christian's personal vocation. In the absence of any reason which definitely either demands or excludes doing something, conscientious discernment is needed to judge whether to do it and how far to go with it. When negative aspects of treatment reach a certain level, the judgment will be to limit it, just as when negative aspects of anything else reach a certain level, it will be limited according to the overall requirements of the patient's personal vocation.

Thus one does not seek care for every little symptom. Urgently needed treatment may be delayed briefly while one meets other important responsibilities. Even in life-threatening situations, one chooses among treatment options in view of the whole of one's responsibilities. These sometimes require that treatment be limited; they also can point to limitation without actually requiring it.

The second way of judging that one may rightly limit medical treatment is by recognizing that one has no desire to go on with it and that no norm requires one to do so. At some point, the burdens of treatment become so great and its benefits so slight that one is not interested in continuing. Of course, the general, affirmative norm that one should seek or continue needed treatment demands that laziness, self-indulgence, and cowardice not prevent one from taking good care of one's life and health. Special responsibilities also may require one to go on with treatment. For example, one might have some important task to complete, or might be impelled by mercy toward those who could benefit from research to accept an experimental treatment. But sometimes there is no such special responsibility and one is confident that laziness, self-indulgence, and cowardice are not behind one's disinclination to go on with treatment. One thus recognizes that nothing requires one to go on with it, and concludes that one may draw the line whenever one feels ready to do so.

The recognition that one has done all that one should to cherish life and health comes most easily when one is certain that one will die soon whether or not one limits treatment. One can be certain of this either because one accepts a confirmed diagnosis that one is suffering from some fatal disease or because one's general condition is so clearly and steadily declining that there is no room for doubt that death is imminent.

But even without being certain that they will die soon in any case, upright people sometimes seem to recognize that they have fulfilled their responsibility to take care of themselves. For example, patients on hemodialysis, who are not doing well and who have no special duty requiring them to go on, sometimes decide to quit treatment. It seems to me that in some cases such a decision is justified, although in others the patient's poor condition is due to lack of self-discipline, and the patient's decision to withraw from the program is due to impatience and faintheartedness.

Whether or not patients are certain they will die soon, their lack of interest in further treatment will be the product of their reflection on both the burdens and the benefits of going on. Potential benefits are not primarily quantitative — simply prolonging life — but qualitative. Patients want restored or preserved functioning, with an opportunity to experience and do things they consider worthwhile. In this sense, quality-of-life considerations are an unavoidable element in any reason which justifies without requiring limitation of treatment.

Those who reject moral absolutes hold that in conflict situations one should commensurate prospective benefits and harms, and choose the option which offers the better proportion of the two. One line of argument against this proportionalism is that the commensuration it requires is impossible. Proportionalists are likely to claim that just such commensuration is admitted in the preceding analysis. However, this claim will be mistaken. The judgment that one is justified in limiting treatment does not override any moral absolute. Rather, this judgment becomes possible only when all relevant moral norms leave open the question of whether or not to limit treatment.

The judgment of conscientious discernment is not a moral judgment reached by commensuration of benefits and harms, considered from a premoral point of view. Rather, patients discern what is suitable for themselves, all things considered; good Christians first consider the total responsibilities of their personal vocation. Thus, the moral standards which shape their commitments and character are operative in their discernment, which leads to a moral judgment only in the sense that it selects what is right for the individual from a set of options all of which are right in themselves.

Similarly, a decision to limit treatment which follows on the recognition that no norm requires that it be continued and that one has no desire to continue with it is a personal choice between morally open alternatives. Prospective benefits and harms are commensurated on the scales of the patient's feelings. When these feelings belong to a virtuous character, whose core is a set of upright commitments faithfully fulfilled, they translate true moral norms into a language which can speak for the individual as a whole, including the bodily self and the subconscious mind. Hence, patients who have fulfilled their responsibilities in respect to treatment are entitled to follow their feelings in choosing from morally open alternatives the option which is right for themselves.

H. The application of the same norms
in making proxy decisions

Sections D-G have clarified the moral norms for limiting medical treatment, assuming they will be applied by patients making judgments for themselves. In itself, the noncompetence of patients to make decisions is irrelevant to what treatment they should get. Moreover, proxies decide rightly if they were both morally upright and able to decide for themselves. Hence, there are no special substantive moral norms to guide proxy judgments.

It is usually easy to make proxy decisions for previously competent patients rendered temporarily noncompetent by some injury or illness. However, anyone making proxy decisions has been competent and expects to be so for some time. Thus, it is hard for proxies to put themselves in the place of the newborn, the irreversibly comatose, and others who have never been competent or will not be so again. Hence, special consideration must be given to some of the problems of proxy decisions to limit treatment for such persons.

In Section D, I explained the concept of direct killing of oneself. If one adopts a proposal to kill oneself and carries out the plan embodied in that proposal, one directly kills oneself. The ulterior reason for adopting the proposal may be good, and the carrying out of its plan can be by limiting treatment. But as long as the proposal is to bring about or hasten death, the act will be suicide. A similar analysis holds true of proposals to bring about or hasten someone else's death. If a proxy chooses to limit treatment so that a patient will die, the withholding of treatment which results in the patient's death is the means of committing murder.

In recent years, many have acknowledged making proxy decisions to limit medical treatment for handicapped infants to ensure their quick death. Morally speaking, the carrying out of such a choice is the direct killing of an innocent person — i.e., murder. A famous case decided by the Indiana Supreme Court exemplifies one class of such murderous proxy decisions to limit medical treatment. An infant afflicted with Down's Syndrome was denied surgery it needed to survive, not because of the burdensomeness of the treatment in comparison with its probable benefit, but simply because the parents did not want a baby with that handicap. In many places, infants who are in no imminent danger of death but are suffering from open spina bifida with a prognosis of severe deformity are selected for so-called nontreatment. "Nontreatment" sometimes means that surgery is omitted, although it might be helpful and is not contraindicated. Of course, if the child nevertheless survives, its handicap is increased. So some are more radical in their "nontreatment:" They withhold feeding, the most basic life-support care, to make sure that the child will die. That clearly is murder.

Does it follow that it is always wrong for proxies to decide that noncompetent patients should not be fed? No. There are times when the ordinary nursing care a good mother gives her child excluded offering the child food. For example, if death is imminent regardless of the care given, and if eating seems only to increase the child's suffering, a good mother would omit feeding but try otherwise to make her child comfortable.

If a patient is not in imminent danger of death but is in an irreversible coma, as the late Miss Karen Quinlan was, life-support care more sophisticated than ordinary nursing care is very costly. It seems to me that such costly care excedes a permanently comatose person's fair share of available facilities and services. Thus, I believe that when Miss Quinlan was removed from intensive care, she ought not to have been placed in a special care facility, but should instead have been sent home or cared for in the hospital with only the sorts of equipment and services available in an ordinary household. These do not include feeding by tube, and Miss Quinlan could not be fed otherwise. Thus, if I am right, she should not have been fed. Not feeding patients in irreversible coma would cause their early death, and it would be wrong to omit feeding them to hasten their death. But a proxy could decide against care in a special nursing facility out of fairness to others, and accept the patient's death as a side effect.

Does it follow that no one is entitled to a lifetime of care, including feeding by tube, at the level Miss Quinlan received? No, because the same principle of fairness by which the cost of that level of care is excessive for people in irreversible coma will require as much or more care for many other patients. This can be seen by applying the Golden Rule, which expresses what fairness demands, to various cases. We all know that each of us might sometime be in irreversible coma, might sometime need public funding of long-term treatment for some other condition, and must always pay taxes. I think we can honestly say that we are willing to limit treatment of ourselves and those we love, if ever in irreversible coma, to ordinary nursing care, without feeding by tube. By setting this limit, we will keep publicly funded special care facilities free for other patients, and avoid increasing taxes to provide additional facilities of this sort. But if we or someone we loved were conscious and able to do some good things and have some good experiences, we would want a lifetime of care at or even above the level Miss Quinlan received, including feeding by tube, if necessary, we would want public funds to be availalbe for what was needed. Hence, we cannot fairly limit others' care if they are in this condition. Nor can we reject the taxation required to provide facilities for such people.

As explained in section G, those convinced they will die soon with or without certain types of treatment often recognize that they have no obligation to prolong their lives as they die. The prospect of the imminent death of non-competent persons should have a similar impact on proxy decisions about their treatment and care. But here there may be a temptation to stretch the meaning of "imminent death" or "terminally ill."

Everyone whose pathological condition is incurable and whose cause of death can be predicted with confidence is dying, yet death may not be imminent. For example, at present everyone suffering from AIDS is dying, but some survive for many months. If death is not imminent, mortal illness is not at its end, and so the patient should not be called "terminally ill." Thus, not everyone who is dying is terminally ill. Patients are terminally ill only when their condition deteriorates steadily, so that it is certain that there will not be even a very brief remission. Because surprising remissions sometimes occur, no one can be sure beyond reasonable doubt that death is imminent — that the patient can be safely considered terminally ill — until death is expected within a few hours or, at most, a few days.

If a patient is permanently noncompetent, terminally ill, and unconscious, an upright proxy may decide to forego all but the ordinary nursing care of a family without special equipment or training could supply in their own home. If such a patient is sometimes conscious, in addition to ordinary nursing care, the proxy should require good palliative care to make the patient comfortable. Thus, in making decisions for such patients, one has no obligation — indeed, it is likely to be morally wrong — to require treatment to resuscitate them, maintain their breathing with respirators, give them blood transfusions, give them food and water intravenously or by tube, fight their infections with antibiotics, and so on, except insofar as such forms of treatment and care may be necessary to ease suffering.

Many people feel intuitively that while it is right not to initiate such forms of treatment and care for terminally ill patients, it is wrong to discontinue them if doing so will lead directly to the patient's death. But, as explained above, the morality of omissions and performances which cause death chiefly hinges on what proposal they carry out and why it is adopted. Thus, if the proposal is to hasten death, either by not initiating or by terminating some sort of treatment or care, the omission or act will be direct killing. But if the proposal is to avoid burdens, and the foreseen patient's death is only accepted as an inevitable side effect, then discontinuing whatever is burdensome is not direct killing, no matter how directly it leads to death. Therefore, any current treatment is justifiably discontinued if its initiation would not now be morally required.

Still, there is a basis in experience for greater reluctance to discontinue life-saving treatment than to omit its initiation. For, at least in the past, decisions not to initiate some potentially life-savings treatment, probably were based on medical contraindications or other burdens, and any act whose foreseeable result was immediate death was an act of violence, outside the context of medical treatment, which carried out a proposal to cause death. But these generalizations based on the sounder morality and simpler technology of earlier days no longer hold true today, when withholding treatment is often advocated as a method of euthanasia and when complex medical technology often becomes excessively burdensome, not least due to its costs, even as it becomes the necessary condition for the survival of terminally ill patients who, with technology of earlier times, would long since have died.

If a patient is permanently noncompetent and dying, but conscious and not terminally ill, the upright proxy often will require treatment needed to prolong life. Most competent, dying persons who are conscious and not terminally ill want life-prolonging treatment, and patients' inability to express their wants should not make any difference. A grave injustice is done dying, noncompetent patients whose treatment is limited simply on the basis that they are dying and noncompetent. For example, if insulin is withheld without a medical contraindication from a noncompetent, dying diabetic, it is clear that this limitation of treatment carries out a proposal to hasten death, since care of this sort neither has itself nor causes any burdens.

Nevertheless, an upright proxy will decide for limitation, if convinced that a conscious and nonterminal patient, if competent, would be justified in limiting treatment, and probably would choose to limit it. Deliberation leading to such a decision, while it must rule out the patient's noncompetence considered in itself, rightly takes into account the difference the patient's noncompetence will make to the burdens and benefits of treatment. For example, a proxy will not require something which cannot succeed without a patient's cooperation when the noncompetent patient's limitations preclude that cooperation. Similarly, if a retarded patient's inability to understand the point of treatment will make it particularly repugnant, that repugnance should be taken into account.

Just as competent patients who are not dying can be justified in limiting medical treatment, so proxies at times may rightly limit it for permanently noncompetent patients do not have serious responsibilities to fulfill, the reasons rooted in such reponsibilities for either requiring or limiting treatment will be irrelevant. But the general, affirmative responsibility to provide needed treatment remains in force. Therefore, withholding from noncompetent patients who are not dying the treatment they need to stay alive cannot be justified unless burdensomeness of one or more kinds is great indeed.

Generally, it is not so great. For example, where the prognosis is good, the burden of surgery to remove cancerous growths is almost never so great that competent people consider refusing such treatment for themselves or those they love. Hence, in cases with a good prognosis, such surgery should be chosen for permanently noncompetent patients, including the severely retarded, the incurably psychotic, and the senile. On the other hand, just as some competent patients on hemodialysis may justifiably withdraw from the program and accept death, so at times a justifiable proxy decision might be made to withdraw from hemodialysis a permanently noncompetent person, whose general condition is poor and whose great repugnance to the treatment is evident.

I. Special norms for the work counselors

Counselors often must help patients and proxies make decisions about medical treatment. This important work has its own moral norms.

Counselors such as priests, who are approached because they hold office in a community, are expected to advise in accord with the community's values and beliefs. If they cannot do so in good conscience, they should either stop counseling or resign their office and offer their services without the community's authorization and support.

Those who counsel about limiting medical treatment should really understand relevant norms and know how to apply them, It is not sufficient to memorize a few rules and follow them blindly, without careful fact-gathering and accurate analysis. For example, it is true that extraordinary means need not be used, and that doubtful laws do not bind. But the abuse of such rules by ill-educated counselors easily leads to unnecessary bodily deaths and spiritual disasters.

The expression, "extraordinary means," signifies those means which are too burdensome in a situation where the reason for wishing to limit care is not a bad one. Means called "extraordinary" in some other sense — e.g., means not usually demanded by the ordinary standard of good medical practice or means which are seldom used — can be obligatory in a particular case. Moreover, no one ever rightly limits treatment in carrying out a proposal to kill or to hasten death. And so, no means excluded with that end in view is morally extraordinary. Therefore, counselors who tell parents of unwanted defective children that they need not consent to life-saving treatment which they would authorise for a wanted child, on the ground that the treatment is in some sense extraordinary, gravely err in applying the rule that extraordinary means need not be used.

The maxim, "Doubtful Laws don't bind," is relevant to moral judgment only in a legalistic framework which is, at best, inadequate. Even within a legalistic framework, the maxim was applicable only after one had done one's best to discover the moral truth. It always was taken for granted that those who enjoy the gift of faith should accept its moral implications as certain and try to live in accord with them. Thus, dissent from very firm and constant moral trachings of the Church never could render these teachings doubtful. And so, counselors abuse legalism if they encourage people to choose arbitrarily between traditional Christian teachings and dissenting theological opinions, by suggesting that the latter make the former doubtful and invoking the maxim that doubtful laws don't bind.

Sometimes people ask moral advisors for help in choosing between two morally acceptable options. In such cases, nondirective counseling techniques are appropriate to help clients clarify their own thoughts and feelings, and so discern which option is right for them. As death approaches and daily choices must be made between morally acceptable options of continuing and limiting treatment, the counselor's moral support often facilitates discernment and inspires the confidence necessary to forestall groundless guilt feelings for making upright but hard choices.

Sometimes counselors are convinced that an option under consideration is morally unacceptable. In many cases, they can uncover appealing aspects of a morally acceptable alternative, or even bring to light a good option which has been entirely overlooked. But whether or not counselors can positively promote upright choices, they must clarify the truth about morally unacceptable alternatives. In doing so, they in no way impose obligations on those they advise. For the counselor's role is neither to make decisions for others nor to give them orders, but to clarify what the counselor says, it is likely to impose itself on the client's conscience. Thus, counselors who try to relieve those they advise of real moral responsibilities are likely both to succeed in encouraging them to make immoral choices and to fail in preventing the grave guilt of those choices.

Finally, counselors who share the light of Christian faith with their clients should make the most of the occasions when they are asked for help in reaching decisions about limiting medical treatment. Generally, such help is sought when life is at stake, and that is a moment of special grace, for it offers a unique opportunity to communicate the gospel effectively. This will be done if the counselor firmly believes that the sufferings of the presnt are unworthy to be compared with the glory for which we hope, clearly communicates this conviction, and unmistakably lives and works according to it. The counselor's living of the gospel makes it credible, when suffering and death at one and the same time test faith and cry out for the light and peace only firm faith can give. Thus, a Christian counselor who lives the gospel truly is another Jesus, who bears others' crosses with them, and so fulfills Jesus' Law — the Law of the cross, the Law of Love.

SELECTED BIBLIOGRAPHY

Ashley, Benedict M., O.P., and Kevin D. O'Rourke, O.P. Health Care Ethics: A Theological Analysis, 2d ed. (St. Louis: The Catholic Health Association of the United States, 1982), 362-88. A chapter in a contemporary Catholic textbook which offers a generally reliable treatment of many of the questions treated in this lecture.

Connery, John R., S.J. "Catholic Ethics: Has the Norm for Rule-Making Changed?" Theological Studies, 42 (1981), 232-50. A critique of proportionalism which clearly shows how far this new morality is from classical Catholic moral theology.

——————, "The Clarence Herbert Case: Was Withdrawal of Treatment Justified?" Hospital Progress, 65 (February 1984), 32-35, 70. An argument for the position, contrary to that presented in the lecture, that it is wrong to withdraw treatment from a patient in irreversible coma.

——————, "The Theology of Proportionate Reason," Theological Studies, 44 (1983), 489-96. An answer to an attempt to reply to his previous article against proportionalism.

Grisez, Germain. "Against Consequentialism," The American Journal of Jusrisprudence and Legal Philosophy, 23 (1978), 21-72. My most complete critique of consequentialism or, as some proponents now call it, proportionalism.

——————— and Joseph M. Boyle, Jr. Life and Death with Liberty and Justice: A Contribution to the Euthanasia Debate (Notre Dame and London: University of Notre Dame Press, 1979. Treats euthanasia and related questions, including those covered in this lecture, but with a focus on jurisprudential problems. Chapter 3 (59-85) deals with the definition of death; chapter 9 (259-97) deals with justice and care for the noncompetent, including infants afflicted with birth defects; chapters 11-12 (336-441) deploy the same ethical theory used in the lecture and apply it to all the relevant issues, but proceed by a strictly philosophical method.

——————, with the help of Joseph M. Boyle, Jr., Basil Cole, O.P., John M. Finnis, John A. Geinzer, Jeannette Grisez, Robert G. Kennedy, Patrick Lee, William E. May, and Russell Shaw. The Way of the Lord Jesus, vol. 1, Christian Moral Principles (Chicago: Franciscan Herald Press, 1983). A full presentation of the fundamental moral theology presupposed in the lecture. Chapter 6 (141-71) treats proportionalism; chapters 7-8 (173-228) treat natural-law principles; chapter 9 (229-49) treats action theory; chapters 19-27 (459-682) treat the purpose of Christian life, the constitution of the Christian as human and divine, and the normative principles of specifically Christian ethics; chapter 35 (831-70) treats the authority of Catholic moral teaching; and chapter 36 (871-916) treats radical theological dissent.

The Linacre Centre for the Study of the Ethics of Health Care. Euthanasia and Clinical Practice: Trends, Principles and Alternatives: The Report of a Working Party (London: The Linacre Centre, 1982). A generally sound and very useful treatment, which gains credibility from the quality and diversity of scholarly expertise brought to the study by the members of the working party. Much of the ground covered in the lecture is treated, but with a focus on euthanasia, jurisprudential issues, and points of view other than that of the patient or proxy making decisions.

McCarthy, Donald G., and Albert S. Moraczewski, O.P., eds. Moral Responsibility in Prolonging Life Decisions (St. Louis: Pope John Center; Chicago: Franciscan Herald Press, 1981). Based on the contributions of fourteen scholars, this volume deals with almost all the questions considered in the lecture. It is generally sound, but chapters vary considerably in quality and usefulness. Most worthwhile are chapter 6 (80-94), on the patient-physician relationship, by Joseph M. Boyle, Jr.; chapter 8 (116-23), on the principles for decisions about prolonging life, by Benedict M. Ashley, O.P.; and chapter 9 (124-38), on the duty of prolonging life and its limits, by John Connery, S.J.

Oden, Thomas C. Should Treatment Be Terminated? Moral Guidelines for Christian Families and Pastors (New York: Harper and Row, 1976). A thoughtful, genuinely Christian treatment by a Protestant theologian, experienced in pastoral counseling. Although I do not agree with everything in this book, I consider it worth careful study for its many insights, and because it is a remarkable witness from outside classical Catholic moral theology to the unity of the Christian tradition.

Ramsey, Paul. The Patient as Person: Explorations in Medical Ethics (New Haven and London: Yale University Press, 1970), 113-64. A thoughtful and influential chapter on the question of limiting care to the terminally ill. Unfortunately, near the end of the chapter (161), Ramsey, a leading Protestant moral theologian whose positions generally conform to the common Christian tradition, suggests that it is justifiable to kill patients who are "irretrievably inaccessible to human care." Noting that it is entirely indifferent to patients at this stage whether they are killed by "an intravenous bubble of air or by the withdrawal of useless ordinary natural remedies such as nourishment," Ramsey overlooks the difference it makes to the decision maker's heart.

Sacred Congregation for the Doctrine of the Faith. "Declaration on Euthanasia," in Vatican Collection, vol 2: Vatican Council II: More Postconciliar Documents, ed. Austine Flannery, O.P. (Northport, N.Y.: Costello Publishing Co., 1982), 510-17. The most recent, authoritative summary of received Catholic teaching on matters treated in the lecture. The lecture is meant to conform to this teaching, and to supply theological clarifications and specifications of many details. Unfortunately, this Declaration was rather weak inasmuch as it did not straightforwardly confront radical theological dissent from the relevant norms it accurately summarized, and so it has been ineffectual in shaping a sounder Catholic response to the antilife movement and present confusion about limiting care.

INDEX